Know About Diabetes

For Insulin-Dependent Diabetics

Dr P.H. Wise PhD, FRCP, FRACP
Consultant Physician
Diabetic and Endocrine Clinic
Charing Cross Hospital, London

W. Foulsham & Co. Ltd.
London · New York · Toronto
Cape Town · Sydney

W. Foulsham & Company Limited
Yeovil Road, Slough, Berkshire, SL1 4JH

ISBN 0-572-01251-9

Filmset in Optima by Filmtype Services Limited,
Scarborough, North Yorkshire and printed at St
Edmundsbury Press, Bury St Edmunds, Suffolk

INTRODUCTION

You may have had diabetes for some time: perhaps you already know much of what is in this book. On the other hand, the diagnosis may have just been made, and all that is involved may seem a little bewildering.

This book was written to give you some idea of what diabetes is all about. It tries to answer the type of questions you will ask, both now and in the future. It cannot cover the whole subject, and at the end you will find a list of books for further reading.

There is one thing upon which most authorities agree: the more that diabetics know, the better controlled and the healthier they are likely to be. Never hesitate to ask for additional information and help.

ACKNOWLEDGEMENTS

The author acknowledges with appreciation the constructive criticism of the many patients, nurses, dietitians and other health professionals who helped to produce this book.

1. WHAT IS DIABETES?

Diabetes is the name given to a disturbed chemical balance in the body, which can affect a number of different organs. The word diabetes comes from a Greek expression meaning "siphon", and refers to the increased urination and thirst which often occurs in newly diagnosed or uncontrolled cases. These symptoms are due to the high sugar (glucose) content in the urine, which in turn follows an excessive build-up of glucose in the blood.

Diabetes is due to partial or complete lack of insulin. This hormone is normally released directly into the blood circulation from small pockets of cells called Islets of Langerhans, which are scattered throughout the pancreas gland (sweetbread). The pancreas rests in the upper abdomen, just beneath the liver, partly behind the stomach in the loop of the duodenum.

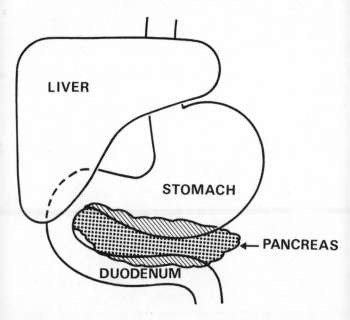

The pancreas also produces enzymes, which pass through a duct into the duodenum, where they assist with digestion of food. This part of the pancreas is only rarely affected in diabetes.

Insulin in usable form was first extracted from animal pancreas in 1921 by two Canadians, Banting and Best. Shortly afterwards it proved successful in the treatment of human diabetes.

About one person in every eighty is diabetic, although only one in four diabetics actually need insulin for treatment.

2. WHAT DOES INSULIN NORMALLY DO?

Insulin has many different effects involving the manufacture of proteins, fats and other substances. However, its main action is to encourage glucose in the blood to enter the cells of all major body tissues, where it is then either stored (as glycogen in the liver and muscle), or used as fuel for almost every chemical process in the body. Therefore, if insufficient insulin is produced, the level of glucose in the blood will rise above normal (hyperglycaemia).

3. HOW DOES UNCONTROLLED DIABETES (HYPERGLYCAEMIA) PRODUCE SYMPTOMS?

When blood glucose rises above normal (see Question 20), a number of things may happen:

a) In the early stages, or if the rise of blood glucose is only moderate, **there may be no symptoms at all**. As the glucose level rises higher, one or more of the following may occur:

b) The lens of the eye may alter its shape, producing **blurring of vision**.

5

c) High glucose levels in the blood reduce the body's defences against infection. Skin, urine, lung and other **infections** may therefore occur. In fact, it may be such an infection which first alerted your doctor that you might have diabetes.

d) By overflowing into the urine (where it is usually first tested) glucose may draw water with it: **more urine** is then passed.

e) Excessive urination reduces the body's fluid reserves and stimulates **thirst** in an attempt to keep body fluid supplies normal.

f) The passing of excessive urine also results in loss of essential chemicals (sodium, potassium and magnesium) producing **cramps**, **tiredness** and **weakness**.

g) Because glucose cannot be properly used by the body and is lost in the urine, the body uses its stores of fat as a fuel supply, resulting in **weight loss**.

h) If very severe loss of fluid occurs, the body becomes dry (**dehydrated**): **breathlessness** and even **coma** may then occur.

4. WHY DOES DIABETES DEVELOP?

There are different types of diabetes, but in most patients the abnormality in insulin production is partly inherited from one or both sides of the family. However, there are almost always additional factors which are responsible for setting the disorder in motion.

In the more late-developing (non-insulin-dependent or maturity-onset) diabetes, insulin deficiency is only mild. In such cases diabetes may show up because of being overweight, or may result from the effects of repeated pregnancy, certain drugs, stress or just ageing itself.

However, in your type of diabetes, whatever your age, the lack of insulin is virtually complete, perhaps resulting from additional severe damage to the pancreas gland by a virus, or due to other factors which we cannot yet identify. Therefore your diabetes is referred to as insulin-dependent or Type I diabetes.

Accordingly, only insulin itself can be used for treatment.

5. DOES DIABETES EVER GO AWAY?

No. It can always be controlled and with treatment you should feel completely well. Even when treated, however, it must still be carefully watched by you and regularly reviewed by your doctor for the rest of your life.

6. WHAT ARE THE MAJOR AIMS AND PRINCIPLES OF DIABETIC TREATMENT?

The first aim of treating your diabetes is to keep your blood glucose level as close as practical to that of a non-diabetic person. By this and other means, the second aim can be achieved: to minimise or avoid the so-called complications of diabetes.

There are three essential principles for achieving these aims: **diet, insulin and exercise**. The diet provides a nutritious source of energy which is reasonably constant from day to day. It must be taken in a pattern which is also predictable throughout each day. This allows it to be accurately matched by the action of insulin, which is usually injected once or twice daily.

Exercise helps to keep body weight constant but in addition lowers the blood glucose level in a very similar way to insulin.

7. HOW IS FOOD NORMALLY PROCESSED BY THE BODY AND WHAT GOES WRONG IN DIABETES?

Foods, which are all different mixtures of carbohydrates, proteins and fats, provide the body with energy. The energy value of any diet is expressed as calories:

> One gram of carbohydrate provides four calories
> One gram of protein provides four calories
> One gram of fat provides nine calories
> One gram of pure alcohol provides seven calories

Food also contains essential minerals and vitamins, but these do not provide the body with usable energy. Depending on age, weight and physical activity the energy needs of the body range between 1000 and 4000 calories per day.

After eating a meal, food passes into the stomach where it is digested (broken down) into smaller particles. Partly digested food then passes into the small intestine where digestion is completed and the small particles pass through the wall of the intestine into the blood stream.

The digested nutrients (carbohydrate, protein and fat) are carried to the liver where they may all be converted into glucose under some circumstances: however, most glucose comes direct from carbohydrate. Consequently, after a meal (especially if it is high in carbohydrate) there is a rise in the amount of glucose in the blood. The following diagram will give you an idea of the normal variation of blood glucose in a non-diabetic person.

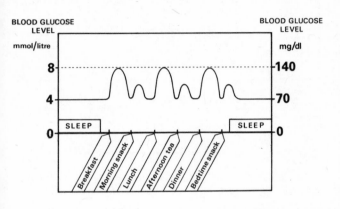

In non-diabetics a rise of blood glucose stimulates the pancreas to produce and release more insulin into the blood vessels which pass through the pancreas. From here, the insulin is distributed to the liver and all other body tissues. In this way, the glucose level is lowered back to normal within two hours by forcing glucose to pass into body cells where it is processed to produce energy. If energy is not needed immediately, insulin allows glucose to be stored in muscles or liver as another carbohydrate called glycogen (to be used when extra energy is needed), or promotes production of fat (for more long-term storage). Insulin also stimulates the formation of proteins, important for the development of muscle, bone and other supporting tissues.

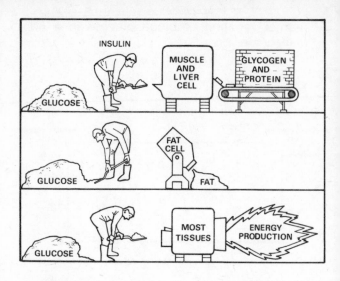

Different tissues use glucose for different purposes

Because diabetics do not produce sufficient insulin, the blood glucose level after a meal remains high and a considerable amount can only be removed from the blood by escaping through the kidneys into the urine. Furthermore, since the body cannot use the glucose properly to produce energy, such energy must be obtained mainly from the breakdown of fat stores and protein-rich tissues in the body. This leads to the loss of weight and ill health of uncontrolled diabetes.

8. WHAT ARE THE PRINCIPLES OF DIABETIC DIETS?

Because carbohydrate foods (sugars and starches such as bread, potatoes, sweets) cause the biggest rise in blood glucose levels, these have been restricted in traditional diabetic diets.

However, research in recent years has shown that although sugar and sugar-containing foods should not be taken (because they need very little digestion and cause rapid rises in blood glucose) we should also be trying to cut down on the amount of fat in the diet.

There are two main reasons for this:

a) All fats (even the vegetable fats and oils found in nuts, cooking oils and margarine) are a very concentrated source of calories and lead to gain in weight if we eat too much of them.

b) Animal fats (as found in eggs, butter, lard, cheese, dripping and meat) are known to increase the chances of developing "hardening of the arteries" (arteriosclerosis) leading to strokes and heart disease.

There are therefore two main rules about diet for all diabetics:

a) Avoid all sugar and sugar-containing foods, and

b) Reduce the amount of fat which you eat, especially from animal sources.

In this way, your diet will include all the more nutritious foods which are required for good health, but will probably contain fewer calories.

Remember that all diabetics have different diets, so that this book cannot provide you with exact guidelines. The amount of food included depends on many factors, including your age, weight and level of activity. Your diet will be designed to suit your way of life, your meal pattern and your likes and dislikes. Consequently a dietitian must spend time with you, drawing up a diet which will suit you as well as helping to control your diabetes.

The dietitian will advise you how many calories and how much and what type of carbohydrate you should have and how to spread your food through the day. It is very important to follow this pattern each day as it is designed to fit in with the type of insulin which you inject. Variation in the amount and timing of the food taken leads to poor diabetic control, unless accompanied by a change of insulin dose or exercise (see Question 14).

High-fibre diets may be of particular benefit to diabetics. Fibre tends to slow down the absorption of other (more refined) carbohydrates from the intestine. It may also level out the swings in blood sugar and occasionally reduce the amount of insulin required. More information is still needed about any long-term advantages. Since many of us (diabetics or not) consume quite a low fibre diet as a result of our high intake of convenience foods, a diet which is high in fibre may well be of benefit to the whole family. Details of high-fibre foods are given at the end of this book.

Your diet will probably be expressed as portions or exchanges, each of which has a content of about 10 grams of carbohydrate. Recognising and learning the portions or exchange values of different foods allows you to vary your food choice. Diabetic diets do not need to be monotonous and uninteresting. Portion or exchange lists for all common foods are given at the end of this book.

Although alcohol is not forbidden to diabetics, it does contain a large number of calories (approximately 7 calories per gram of pure alcohol). Some alcoholic drinks also contain a lot of carbohydrate, so do ask the dietitian for advice on the amount and type of alcohol you may have.

Drinking alcohol, particularly on an empty stomach, can also produce a serious lowering of blood glucose: hypoglycaemia. This is due to a unique chemical action of alcohol itself, so that you should always eat with your drink! (see Question 23).

- 1 pint of beer or dry cider contains about 200 calories
- 1 pub measure of spirits ($1\frac{1}{2}$ fluid ounces) contains about 100 calories
- 1 glass of dry wine contains about 100 calories
  – and remember to count in the mixers too!

It is very important to see a dietitian regularly: you will be given a lot of information and no-one would expect you to remember it all at your first visit. Furthermore, the diet may need to be changed over a period of time – particularly if you change your way of life, gain weight or if the type of insulin you use is changed. Check with Question 38 to be sure you have a contact number for your dietitian.

9. HOW IS INSULIN GIVEN?

Insulin is a complex protein which is mostly extracted from either beef or pig pancreas. However, it is now possible to produce synthetic human insulin on a commercial scale, although there is at present no good evidence that human insulin has any long term benefits compared with purified beef or pork insulin. Insulin needs to be injected, because if taken by mouth the digestive enzymes of the stomach and intestine destroy it before it can be absorbed.

The amount of insulin used in treatment is expressed in units. Throughout the world insulin is

manufactured in various strengths (concen
trations). 40 or 80 units per millilitre (ml) is used
in most European countries and 100 units per m
in the USA, Canada, Australia and most recently
in the UK and Ireland.

It is important to check your insulin each time i
is prescribed and dispensed, to make sure tha
you have both the correct strength and type. I
should always be kept cool (but never frozen)
preferably in a domestic refrigerator.

10. WHAT ARE THE DIFFERENCES BETWEEN THE VARIOUS TYPES OF INSULIN?

Soluble (clear, regular) insulin consists of the pure
hormone whose action has not been prolonged
by any additive. A number of equally short-acting
insulins are available of either beef (bovine) or pig
(porcine) origin. Their length of action depends
on the dose given but is rarely longer than 8–10
hours, so that two or sometimes even three injec
tions need to be given each day to adequately
control the blood glucose level. The higher the
dose, the greater and more prolonged the effec
on blood glucose, and the same applies to all the
other types of insulin described later.

Insulin can be linked to various proteins which
prolong its action to between 14 and 34 hours
depending on the type and dose used. By
contrast, these long-acting insulins are usually
cloudy and mostly need be given only once a
day. Some insulins are biphasic (mixture of shor
and long-acting insulins) and provide better
control on a single dose daily in the majority o
cases.

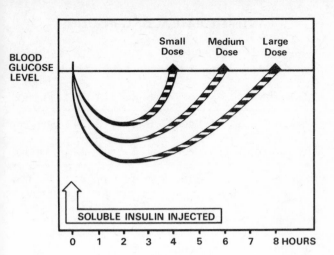

SHORT-ACTING INSULINS

Name	Animal of Origin	Peak (Hrs)	Duration (Hrs)	Purity
Soluble	Beef	3–4	6–10	Standard
Actrapid MC/ Human	Pork/ Syn hum	3–4	6–10	Highly Purified
Hypurin Neutral	Beef	3–5	6–8	Purified
Velosulin/ Human	Pork/ Syn hum	2–3	6–8	Highly Purified
Neusilin	Beef	3–5	6–9	Purified
Humulin S	Syn hum	2–3	6–10	Highly Purified
Quicksol	Beef	3–4	6–10	Purified

15

INTERMEDIATE-ACTING INSULINS

Semilente	Beef	4–6	12–16	Standard
Semitard MC	Pork	6–8	14–16	Highly Purified
Isophane	Beef	6–8	18–24	Standard
Hypurin Isophane	Beef	6–8	18–22	Purified
Insulatard	Pork	5–8	20–24	Purified
Protaphane	Syn hum	6–8	18–24	Highly Purified
Neuphane	Beef	7–8	24–28	Purified
Globin	Beef	8–10	20–24	Standard
Lente	Beef	8–12	22–30	Standard
Hypurin Lente	Beef	8–10	22–30	Purified
Lentard MC	Beef/Pork	8–12	22–26	Highly Purified
Monotard MC	Pork	8–12	20–24	Highly Purified
Neulente	Beef	8–10	24–28	Purified
Rapitard MC	Pork/Beef	4–10	16–20	Highly Purified
Mixtard/Human	Pork/ Syn hum	4–6	20–24	Highly Purified
Initard/Human	Pork/ Syn hum	4–6	20–24	Highly Purified
Humulin I	Syn hum	6–8	18–24	Highly Purified
Human Monotard	Syn hum	8–12	20–24	Highly Purified

Monophane	Beef	8–10	18–22	Purified
Tempulin	Beef	8–12	22–30	Purified

LONG-ACTING INSULINS

Protamine Zinc (PZI)	Beef	14–16	28–34	Standard
Hypurin Protamine Zinc	Beef	14–16	28–34	Purified
Ultralente	Beef	10–18	28–34	Standard
Ultratard MC	Beef	10–18	28–34	Highly Purified

Your doctor may prescribe twice daily injections of short-acting, biphasic or long-acting insulin, since there is evidence that this provides better control for many diabetics. It certainly allows a more flexible approach to your life-style, since each dose can be varied according to changes in exercise and food intake.

Many insulins are now available in a purified form which may have some advantages. The ability to minimise and even reverse fatty changes at sites of injection is the only currently proven advantage of these insulins. Other benefits may emerge in due course.

Although different manufacturers produce very similar insulins, once control has been achieved it is important to keep to the same manufacturer since minor differences may cause you to react differently. Always check the insulin carefully as soon as it has been dispensed by your pharmacy, since dispensing errors can occur.

11. AT WHAT TIMES SHOULD INSULIN BE GIVEN?

Insulin should always be injected 20–30 minutes before breakfast (and also before the evening meal if twice daily insulin is being given). The interval between the injection and the meal should be kept as constant as possible. Too early an injection may result in blood glucose levels falling too low before food is absorbed into the blood stream: this is particularly important when short-acting insulins are being used. Too late an injection may result in blood glucose rising too high before the insulin has a chance to act. Both situations are clearly undesirable.

12. HOW DO I MANAGE SYRINGES AND INJECTIONS?

Syringes are either glass or plastic disposable, now almost universally fitted with Luer-type or fixed needles. Many people find the disposable plastic syringes preferable, although their convenience can be outweighed by slightly greater cost over a period of time. Disposable needles are now almost standard.

Many doctors feel that a disposable syringe can be re-used quite safely, but check with yours to be sure he agrees with this approach. If so, after injection replace the syringe in its plastic envelope without rinsing it and keep it in the refrigerator. Every week a new syringe and needle should be used, although blunting of the needle may mean changing it more frequently.

A glass syringe should be rinsed and left in industrial quality spirit (isopropyl alcohol), not surgical spirit which can contain minor impurities. This should be changed each week. The Diabetic Association office can provide you with a special travelling kit in which glass syringes can be kept.

Syringes vary both in capacity (1 ml or 2 ml) and in markings, which can be confusing. You should always confirm with your doctor or nurse exactly how the marks on the syringe correspond to the dose to be injected. The standard ½ ml syringe provides 1 unit for every mark: the 1 ml syringe provides 2 units for every mark.

A) Drawing up Insulin

1) Clean the rubber cap of the insulin ampoule with spirit.
2) Disperse any surplus spirit in the syringe by pulling plunger in and out several times.
3) Draw back the same amount of air into the syringe as the quantity of insulin you will need to draw up.
4) Inject the air into the ampoule.
5) Slowly draw back the quantity of insulin required. If an air space or bubbles develop, move plunger in and out until correct amount of insulin, free of bubbles, is in the syringe. Then withdraw the needle.

Different types of short- and long-acting insulins are sometimes prescribed to be given at the same time. Mostly, they can be mixed safely in the same syringe prior to injection. In this case draw up the clear insulin first, then the cloudy, and inject as soon as possible.

Some insulin combinations have their actions altered by such mixing. Check with your doctor to see if your insulins are "non mixers". If so, give one type first, detach the syringe from the needle (which is left in the skin) and draw up the second type. Then re-attach the syringe to the needle and inject again.

B) Injection Technique (which will be demonstrated by the doctor or nurse)

1) You may clean the skin with spirit before giving an injection. However, if you bathe regularly and keep yourself clean this is not strictly necessary. Spirit tends to toughen the skin, making injections more difficult and makes your needles blunt more quickly.

2) Injections should be given under the skin, not into it, using a needle no longer than ½" (1.2 cm). The injection should ideally be given vertically, but certainly at no smaller angle than 45°, and the needle almost inserted to the hilt.

3) Withdraw the plunger very slightly just before injecting the insulin, to be certain that you have not accidentally entered a blood vessel. Also be sure, especially with glass syringes, that there is no leakage of insulin around the plunger while injecting.

4) Never use exactly the same spot twice in succession, although different spots no closer than 2–3 cm (1" apart) in the same area can be used successfully. Ideally rotate the injection sites so that a different major area is used for each injection. Repeated injections in the same area are more likely to produce swelling (hypertrophy) or loss (atrophy) of fat tissues at the site of the injection. However, the recently available pure insulins (see Question 10) are less likely to cause these problems. Furthermore, transferring to these purified insulins can cause any atrophy or hypertrophy already present to become less obvious or even disappear.

5) Some stinging during the injections is usual; pain or burning after the injection, or irritation or reddening at the site of the injection are abnormal and should lead to discussion with your doctor. The cause may be either faulty injection technique or an allergy to the type of insulin being used.

6) When going to your doctor or the pharmacy always take both a syringe and an empty insulin package or ampoule with you, to compare with what is being newly prescribed or supplied. This will help to avoid errors.

C) Placing of Injections

Every diabetic develops his or her personal routine, but the diagram below shows the range of possibilities.

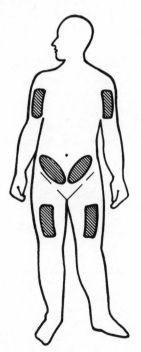

In some people insulin seems to have a more rapid effect if injected into the arms than the legs, with a slower effect still from the wall of the abdomen. Your own experience may lead to the use of certain areas rather than others.

13. IS EXERCISE IMPORTANT?

Yes. Any form of exercise causes the muscles to use more glucose. Not only is the blood glucose level lowered immediately after exercise, but there appears to be a long-term lowering of blood glucose in people whose life-style is more energetic. Taking exercise often means that you should reduce your insulin dose beforehand – or increase your intake of food.

Most people do not realise how inactive they really are. Tiredness and fatigue after a day's work are due more to emotional stress and tension than to the effects of muscular exercise.

Any type of exercise is satisfactory for diabetics including cycling, regular sport or just plain walking. A careful look at your life-style and discussion with friends and family should help you plan a more energetic way of life, whatever your age or other medical problems.

Remember that many factors can affect the blood glucose level and the following diagram will remind you of the most important ones.

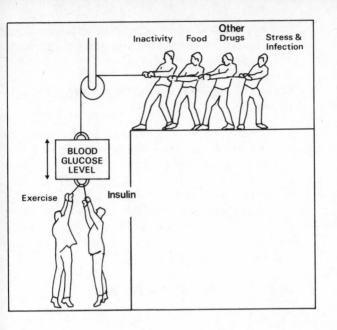

14. CAN EXERCISE PROVIDE ANY PROBLEMS?

Yes. If both food intake and insulin dose remain the same, a sudden increase in exercise can result in quite a sudden fall of blood glucose, producing an insulin reaction (hypoglycaemia or "hypo"). The symptoms of this will be described later in this booklet (see Question 22). It can be prevented by:

a) Eating a larger meal before, or nibbling during exercise.

b) Reducing the insulin dose on the morning (or evening) of planned exercise (eg. game of squash) by a proportion which your doctor will advise, or you will work out yourself by trial and error.

c) Always carrying lumps or cubes of sugar (or a glucose tablet such as Dextrosol) with you in case a "hypo" occurs, or to prevent one should the exercise prove longer and more severe than anticipated.

15. WHAT IS THE "HONEYMOON" PHASE OF DIABETES?

In some diabetics, the insulin dose needed to control blood glucose falls during the first few weeks or months of treatment. Occasionally insulin needs to be stopped altogether. However, this is only temporary and does not indicate that your diabetes is cured. Watch your urine or blood tests carefully and be prepared to recommence the insulin. The cause of this interesting phenomenon is still not clear.

16. WHY CONTROL DIABETES WELL?

It is not difficult to provide a pattern of diet, insulin and exercise in such a way as to avoid the symptoms of both hyperglycaemia (Question 3) and hypoglycaemia (Question 23) but this is not enough!

Particularly if you are young, with a long life span ahead, keeping blood glucose levels as close as possible to those of a non-diabetic appears to reduce the likelihood of getting the so-called complications of diabetes in later life. These are dealt with in Question 29.

Achieving good control requires a lot of your own involvement and thought, and your doctor will be glad to provide additional guidelines on the many small ways through which control can be improved.

17. HOW CAN YOU TELL WHETHER YOUR DIABETES IS WELL CONTROLLED?

By the way you feel? No! This can be most unreliable. Many diabetics may feel perfectly well despite having uncontrolled diabetes: yet such a situation can produce undesirable effects over a period of time. The symptoms listed in Question 3 should be well recognised by you: if they occur, your diabetes is badly out of control! The cause must be found and corrected immediately.

By testing the urine? Yes! Every insulin-receiving diabetic should test their urine (or blood) once or more each day.

By testing the blood? Yes! Measuring the blood glucose is becoming more simple. It can of course be accurately done in the laboratory. In addition, strips are available (Visidex or BM 20–800) which, when covered by a drop of blood obtained by pricking your own finger or ear lobe, change colour according to the blood glucose level.

Small, pocket-size and comparatively inexpensive meters are also available to measure this colour change and measure blood glucose rather more accurately. These techniques enable you yourself to assess and control your own diabetes to a degree which was previously impossible. Your doctor will be happy to discuss these procedures with you.

Untreated or poorly controlled diabetes also raises the blood level of certain fats (lipids) including cholesterol and triglyceride. Your doctor may check the blood levels of these fats from time to time and may advise a change in diet if they are abnormal. There is considerable evidence to suggest that keeping blood fats at normal levels improves the long-term health of arteries (see Question 29).

A more recently introduced blood test (called haemoglobin A1) provides an estimate of average blood glucose over the previous days or weeks, and helps your physician to assess yet another aspect of control. More tests of this type are being gradually introduced into clinical use.

18. HOW IS URINE TESTED FOR GLUCOSE?

A number of ways have been developed.

Clinistix (or Testape). These dip-strips are useful only for finding out whether glucose is present or not: they are not satisfactory for assessing the actual amount, and should not be used routinely by diabetics.

Diabur-5000 or Diastix dip-strips show a better and more definite colour change, depending on how much glucose is present. These are satisfactory for routine use. The result should be recorded as 0, 1/10, 1% etc.

Ketodiastix, which enables you to measure ketone levels on the same "dip" are also available (see Question 25).

Clinitest tables (to which 5 drops of urine and 10 drops of water are added in a test tube) provide a similar range of colours. These are also satisfactory and possibly a little more accurate than Diastix. The result is recorded as 0, 1/4, 1/2% etc. to a maximum of 2%. A "2-drop test" (using 2 drops of urine and 10 drops of water) can be used: this allows measurement of urine glucose levels right up to 5%. However a different colour chart must be used.

Whichever test you use, it is important that you very carefully follow the instructions which accompany the test kit: the length of the "dip" and the time at which you "read" the colour are both of the utmost importance.

Aspirin (in doses of more than 600 mg per day) or Vitamin C (in doses of more than 250 mg per day) can affect the chemicals in the urine testing equipment. They can reduce the apparent sugar when using strips, and raise the apparent sugar when using Clinitest.

19. WHEN SHOULD URINE BE TESTED?

Before meals is the least likely time to show glucose; one to two hours after meals is usually the most likely time to show glucose. Your doctor will recommend one or both times and probably suggest a bedtime test as well on certain evenings. The object of urine testing is to obtain a clear picture of your control during the waking hours, and 2 to 4 tests a day are usually necessary to provide this picture for you and your doctor.

Testing during the working day is useful, although possibly inconvenient. However, you can pass a sample into a small clean bottle (such as a well washed out tablet bottle), and test it when you get home later in the day.

The urine that you test has been produced by the kidneys during the period since you last emptied your bladder; the early morning test therefore gives no information about control at that time, but only gives an idea of the average control through the previous night.

To deal with this problem, "second sample" or "interval" testing is often recommended. In this procedure, urine is passed at say 7.00 am then again at 7.30 am, only the second sample being tested. This gives a better reflection of the blood glucose at that particular time. The same procedure can obviously be used at other times of the day.

It is essential that you write down all your test results in a test record book and bring it to the clinic or doctor's surgery at each visit. In this way he or she can see exactly how you are getting on and can perhaps help you improve your control. Without this information, your doctor can only give a fraction of the help that would otherwise be possible.

20. WHAT IS A NORMAL BLOOD GLUCOSE LEVEL?

In people without diabetes, fasting blood glucose (after not eating overnight) is less than 5 millimoles per litre or 90 milligrams per decilitre (shortened to mmol/l or mg/dl). After food it rarely rises above 8 mmol/l (145 mg/dl). In untreated or uncontrolled diabetes, blood glucose may even rise above 30 mmol/l (540 mg/dl).

With treatment your doctor will aim to keep your level at less than 10 mmol/l (180 mg/dl) for all or most of the time, and will in many cases help you to achieve the lower, more normal, levels mentioned above. It is important to emphasise that symptoms of hyperglycaemia (Question 3) rarely occur unless blood glucose is consistently higher than 14 mmol/l (250 mg/dl). **Therefore just because you feel well, it does not necessarily indicate that your diabetes is controlled.**

21. DO POSITIVE GLUCOSE TESTS IN THE URINE ALWAYS INDICATE POOR CONTROL?

No! The amount of glucose which appears in the urine depends not only on blood glucose levels but also on the height of the kidney barrier to the "overflow" of glucose. It may help to compare this process to the function of a storage tank.

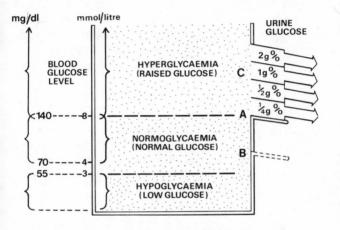

In non-diabetics, glucose rarely appears in the urine because this kidney barrier or "threshold" is normally 8–10 mmol/l (145–180 mg/dl: A in Figure) and as indicated earlier, blood glucose of a non-diabetic does not usually exceed this figure.

The threshold is also normal (8–10 mmol/l) in many diabetics, so that absence of urine glucose *usually* means that the blood glucose is not above this level.

Some diabetics, however, have a low threshold for glucose (B in Figure), occasionally even as low as 4 mmol/l (70 mg/dl). This means that glucose overflows into the urine even with a normal blood glucose level. Should the urine be then kept free of glucose all the time, you are almost certainly overtreating the diabetes with a real risk of producing hypoglycaemia. Pregnancy almost always produces a low threshold, so that urine tests become particularly unreliable as a means of assessing control in this situation.

On the other hand, some diabetics, particularly with increasing age or kidney disorder, have a high threshold (C in Figure). Blood glucose can then be quite high, without glucose appearing in the urine, giving a false impression of good control.

By regularly comparing blood glucose and urine glucose, your doctor will check your threshold from time to time. It is your responsibility to know exactly what your threshold is, and therefore what significance you can attach to glucose being present in the urine in your own particular case.

Measurement of blood glucose by one of the self-testing methods mentioned in Question 17 is particularly useful where the threshold is abnormal.

22. HOW CAN I ACHIEVE THE BEST POSSIBLE CONTROL OF MY DIABETES?

This is probably one of the most important questions for an insulin-dependent diabetic to ask! It is not easy because our lifestyle varies so much during a single day, and from one day to the next. A normal pancreas adjusts to diet, exercise and stress automatically by changing its output of insulin. Being diabetic, *you* have to take over this function.

Firstly, always have three regular meals each day, with an early morning, mid-afternoon and before-bedtime snack. If you go out for a meal which might be larger than usual, it doesn't hurt once in a while, but **anticipate** by taking more insulin beforehand. Being prepared to do finger-tip blood sugar tests after such an unusual meal will tell you whether you have adjusted your dose correctly. Remember that half an hour after a meal, blood glucose should not exceed 10 mmol/l (180 mg/dl). The same **anticipation** applies to stress situations (examinations, performances, arguments, as well as infections of all types): don't wait for diabetes to go out of control, raise the dose first.

If you measure your blood glucose level often enough, you will learn to judge how much more insulin than usual you need for such situations.

The same **anticipation** is the keynote to handling exercise (see also Question 14). Drop your insulin dose by anything from 4 units to half of your usual dose before a game of tennis, a long hike or a cycle ride. Taking extra carbohydrate with exercise may of course suit you better. Always check your blood glucose level to see whether you have done it correctly.

Remember that on two doses of insulin each day, your morning dose affects the blood glucose at midday and before the evening meal, while your evening dose affects the late night and early morning glucose levels. Achieve before-meal blood glucose levels of 4–7 mmol/l (70–120 mg/dl) and immediate after-meal levels of 7–10 mmol/l (120–180 mg/dl) and you can be very pleased with yourself.

Blood testing at home isn't necessarily a routine for everybody. But if you do it, there should be considerable attention to detail. Whether you use the blood strip tests alone (checking colour change against a chart) or with one of the many meters currently available, the result that you get depends very much on the following points of technique:

a) Always ensure that you prick your finger deeply enough to get a free flow of blood (milking the finger does not produce a good sample). Use one of the commercially-available lancets with or without an automatic pricking device and consider the use of the edge of the palm or your knuckles if your finger-tips are getting too sore.

b) Place a "blob" of blood on the test strip pad: not a smear!

c) Pay particular attention to the timing instructions given by the makers of the strip. Even a few seconds out could give you an incorrect result.

d) Do you use a meter?

   1) If not self-calibrating, check calibration before each test.
   2) If it is self-calibrating (the better type of meter), it is still a good idea to use a test strip with a known blood glucose concentration before you read your own result, just to be sure that the meter is working correctly.
   3) The "window" of the meter can get dirty. Follow the maker's instructions carefully as to how, and how often, you should clean it.

Even if you get the most accurate blood glucose

result, it will only improve your control if you act on it! Therefore do at least one or two tests a day, record the results together with any unusual happenings (such as insulin reactions) in your test record book, and be prepared to adjust, as outlined above, the various aspects of your lifestyle. Contact your doctor or nurse as often as you think necessary. Do not wait until your next appointment before getting this advice, otherwise you will have lost valuable time in terms of the health of your body.

23. WHAT IS HYPOGLYCAEMIA (INSULIN REACTION OR "HYPO")?

When the blood glucose level falls below 3 mmol/l (55 mg/dl) the following symptoms may develop:

hunger	dizziness
sweating	faintness
palpitations	confusion and vagueness
trembling	loss of consciousness
slurring of speech	and fits

A "hypo" occurring at night may reveal itself only by restlessness, nightmares, and a headache the morning-after. A positive ketone but negative glucose test in the first urine passed next morning is another possible clue to a "hypo" occurring during the previous night.

Every diabetic has a slightly different pattern of symptoms of hypoglycaemia: in fact your doctor may deliberately arrange to give you a "hypo" to help you recognise the symptoms, should they later occur.

The main causes of hypoglycaemia are:

a) Late or missed meals.
b) Accidental overdose of insulin.

33

c) Increased physical activity, without an increase in food or a decrease in insulin.

d) Drinking alcohol on an empty stomach.

Hypoglycaemia is therefore a preventable problem.

a) Late or missed meals should never occur, and the risks of hypoglycaemia are much reduced by ensuring that you have three proper meals together with a mid-morning, mid-afternoon and bedtime snack. Sugar or "Dextrosol" in your pocket or purse will also help to avoid this problem in an emergency.

b) Accidental overdose of insulin, if it does occur, can usually be dealt with by taking extra carbohydrate. However if you realise that an accidental overdose has been given which exceeds the usual dose by more than half, contact your doctor immediately for advice.

c) Increased physical activity may not always be predictable, making it essential to have lump sugar, a Dextrosol tablet or something similar at hand at all times (see Question 14).

d) When drinking alcohol (especially spirits), ensure that you eat at the same time.

The body has efficient built-in mechanisms for reversing mild to moderate hypoglycaemia, but these should never be relied upon to correct this abnormal situation. Repeated attacks of severe hypoglycaemia can result in brain damage. Therefore, the occurrence of frequent hypoglycaemia should immediately be mentioned to your doctor so that changes in insulin or diet can be carried out.

24. HOW SHOULD HYPOGLYCAEMIA BE TREATED?

Firstly, avoid hypoglycaemia where possible. Always have lump (cube) sugar or Dextrosol in your pocket or handbag to correct minor hypoglycaemia should it occur. More severe hypoglycaemia should be promptly corrected by an immediate snack of sweetened milk and a biscuit (or cookie). Should you become drowsy and unable to take action yourself, your identification bracelet or pendant should enable others to provide forced-feeding with a sweetened drink.

Failing this, a doctor will need to give you a glucose injection directly into a vein, and if no doctor is immediately on hand, no time should be wasted in having you transferred to the emergency department of the nearest hospital. From this point of view family, friends, employers or other working colleagues should be made aware of the action they should take under such circumstances.

Glucagon, a hormone which has the opposite effect to insulin, is also available. If you tend to get severe episodes of hypoglycaemia, particularly if you live remote from medical care, your doctor may supply ampoules of glucagon to be given to you in an emergency by a relative or friend. The usual dose is 1 mg (in 1 ml of solution) given in exactly the same way as insulin.

25. WHAT ARE KETONES AND HOW DOES ONE TEST FOR THEM?

Body fat is nothing more than an insulator and a reserve store of energy. If a person eats nothing for 12–18 hours, fat is broken down to provide this reserve energy. Some of the breakdown products of fat are substances called ketones, and these will appear in the urine under such circumstances, whether a person is a diabetic or not.

In the diabetic however, ketones will also appear in the urine if diabetes goes badly out of control. This occurs because there is not enough insulin to provide the body cells with the energy (glucose) that they need: here again the reserve energy (fat) stores are being called upon.

This is a serious warning!

Ketones are tested by Acetest tablets or Ketostix strips (which are just as accurate) and can usually be provided as the combined Keto-diastix strips so that glucose and ketones can be measured at the same time.

26. WHAT ARE KETOACIDOSIS AND DIABETIC COMA?

If diabetic control remains poor, ketones cannot be rapidly enough excreted in the urine, and ketone levels will rise in the blood as well. Because ketones are acids, this affects the entire bodily function, and tiredness, drowsiness, sickness and vomiting can occur. In addition, by this time the large amount of glucose in the urine will cause an excessive loss of water. The mouth becomes dry, breathing becomes deep and rapid and if no action is taken coma develops.

This whole sequence rarely occurs in less than 24 hours, so that there is time to take avoiding action. Before the days of insulin, ketoacidosis was the major cause of death in diabetics. Today, provided ketoacidosis is identified and treated early, recovery is the rule. However, ketoacidosis is preventable.

Taking Action!

If you are thirsty or passing more urine than usual, or show heavy (2%) urine glucose (or blood glucose over 20 mmol/l) at any time, you should immediately check for ketones. If positive, test the urine again in four hours. If still present, you must immediately contact your clinic, hospital or family doctor unless you have been given other specific instructions on dealing with this situation (see Question 37, "Hotline").

27. HOW CAN KETOACIDOSIS BE PREVENTED?

There is always good reason for the loss of control which leads to ketoacidosis:
Too much food or too little exercise.
Too little insulin (forgotten or incorrect dose).
Some medications such as cortisone-like drugs, water tablets (diuretics) etc.
Infection or other stress.

a) **Food and exercise problems.** These are easily prevented by either avoiding changes in eating and exercise patterns, or increasing the dose of insulin before problems arise. By how much should you increase the insulin is a matter of trial-and-error.

b) **Your requirements of insulin** can change over a period of time. Showing consistently higher sugar should prompt you to either increase the dose of insulin slightly (2–8 units) or preferably contact your doctor.

A forgotten insulin dose is not a catastrophe: if you remember before your midday meal, give half to two-thirds your usual dose. If you only remember before your evening meal give one-third to one-half your usual morning dose and make sure you have an extra 20–30 grams (2–3 portions or exchanges) of carbohydrate before retiring. If in doubt contact your doctor or clinic immediately.

c) **Additional drugs** which you are prescribed should always be discussed with your physician to ensure that they do not interfere with diabetic control. Furthermore, certain tablets (such as aspirin and vitamin C) interfere with the chemical reactions in both Diastix and Clinitest tablets although they do not actually affect the glucose content of blood or urine. Therefore, if you are taking these preparations regularly, you may get a mistaken idea of your diabetic control (see Question 18).

d) **Infection and stress** are unavoidable aspects of life. Any stress, whether physical (an accident), mental (worry or depression) or medical (operations, infections or even a common cold) will cause some rise in blood glucose level to an extent which differs from person to person. In any of these situations, the insulin may need to be raised by anything from 4 units to double the usual dose as soon as (or preferably before) urine or blood glucose level indicates a loss of control. You will get to know your own responses to these stresses, and discussion with your doctor will help to provide additional guidelines.

If your illness makes you vomit, feel sick or you cannot eat, do not stop your insulin, continue the same dose: it may even need to be raised. Try to keep taking fluids which also provide some carbohydrate. The following foods may be useful if you are unwell because they provide concentrated carbohydrate in a liquid form to balance the effect of the insulin you are taking.

Food	Amount	
Sugar	2 teaspoons	10 g/½ oz
Glucose	2 teaspoons	10 g/½ oz
Jam/Honey/Marmalade	2 teaspoons	14 g/½ oz
Ribena (undiluted)	1 tablespoon	16 ml
Orange squash (undiluted)	2 tablespoons	35 ml
Orange juice	½ cup	105 ml/4½ fl.oz
Coca-Cola	1 small glass	95 ml/4 fl.oz
Lemonade	1 glass	178 ml/7 fl.oz
Bournvita/Ovaltine/ Drinking Chocolate	2 teaspoons	13 g/½ oz
Milk pudding (tinned)	3 tablespoons	68 g/2¾ oz
Complan (powder)	1 tablespoon	20 g/¾ oz
Build-Up (powder)	½ sachet	15 g/½ oz

If ketones appear, contact the "hotline" number immediately (see Question 37). If you remain ill as long as six hours arrange for someone to take you to the closest hospital accident and emergency (casualty) department at once.

28. IS WEIGHT CONTROL IMPORTANT?

Yes. Being overweight increases your need for insulin and can make your diabetes less stable. It may also cause or aggravate conditions unrelated to diabetes such as high blood pressure and arthritis.

The only way you can influence your weight is by diet and exercise (see Question 13). Remember that one extra hour of brisk walking (or half-an-hour of continuous swimming, jogging or squash) each day will almost predictably allow you to lose about 7 kgs (15 pounds) in a year – providing you do not increase your food intake! Use the table overleaf as a guide to your goal weight.

A weight 2–2.5 kgs (5 pounds) above or below the "desirable" is acceptable!

ADULT DESIRABLE WEIGHT

| HEIGHT (without shoes) | | WEIGHT (without clothes) | | | |
| | | MEN | | WOMEN | |
Feet/ Inches	Centi- metres	Pounds	Kilo- grams	Pounds	Kilo- grams
4/10	147.5	—	—	107	48.5
4/11	150.0	—	—	110	50.0
5/0	152.5	—	—	113	51.5
5/1	155.0	—	—	116	52.5
5/2	157.5	129	58.5	119	54.0
5/3	160.0	133	60.5	122	55.5
5/4	162.5	136	62.0	126	57.0
5/5	165.0	139	63.0	130	59.0
5/6	167.5	143	65.0	135	61.0
5/7	170.0	147	66.5	139	63.0
5/8	172.5	152	69.0	143	65.0
5/9	175.5	156	71.0	147	66.5
5/10	178.0	160	72.5	151	68.5
5/11	180.5	165	75.0	155	70.5
6/0	183.0	170	77.0	—	—
6/1	185.5	175	79.5	—	—
6/2	188.0	180	81.5	—	—
6/3	190.5	185	83.5	—	—
6/4	193.0	190	86.0	—	—

29. WHAT ARE THE SO-CALLED COMPLICATIONS OF DIABETES?

Arteriosclerosis (hardening of the arteries) occurs to some extent in almost every person as they age, whether they are diabetic or not. In some diabetics, it may occur somewhat earlier than usual. Arteriosclerosis is the cause of stroke and heart attacks. It may also produce poor circulation in the legs which leads to painful calves on walking, ulcers on the feet and occasionally gangrene. Keeping to your diet and the avoidance of smoking are both very important in helping to prevent this problem.

Cataracts are degenerative changes in the lens of the eye which can cause dimness of vision. Cataracts occur commonly in non-diabetics and somewhat more frequently in diabetics.

Retinopathy is the name given to leaky and abnormally fragile small blood vessels in the retina, the seeing part of the eye. Such abnormalities may cause blurring, and occasionally loss of vision.

It is the retina that the doctor is examining when he looks in your eyes with an ophthalmoscope.

Blurring of vision is, however, more often due to a change in the shape of the lens because of a rise or fall in the blood glucose level, in which case the blurring tends to vary from hour to hour or from day to day. If blurring persists, see your doctor promptly.

Neuropathy signifies nerve damage, which can cause weakness, pins and needles or a loss of feeling in the hands or feet and occasionally dizziness and other unusual symptoms. Even a lack of sexual performance can occur, although this is more often due to factors other than diabetes.

Nephropathy means kidney damage, which may occur after long-standing diabetes. It is for this reason that your doctor checks for protein in your urine when you visit him and if present it may be an early sign of this problem, although there are many other causes.

Infection, particularly of the skin and urinary system, is more likely to occur in diabetics than in people without diabetes. In addition, healing of even minor injuries is sometimes slower.

All these complications can be effectively treated, particularly if detected early. It is for this reason that the doctor will make a systematic examination of various parts of your body approximately once each year. Keeping your diabetes well-controlled is also one way that you yourself can help reduce the risk of these complications.

30. DOES EVERY DIABETIC GET COMPLICATIONS AT SOME TIME?

No. There is good evidence that most of the above complications are less likely to occur if the diabetes is well-controlled and if weight gain is avoided. However, it must be admitted that even the best controlled diabetic sometimes does have one or other of the complications mentioned above.

31. HOW IMPORTANT IS FOOT CARE?

A diabetic's feet can be very vulnerable. Nerve damage (neuropathy) can prevent feeling an injury, scratch or cut; poor blood supply to the feet may then mean poor healing of the injury and infection or gangrene can develop.

The following rules are important to follow:

a) Avoid walking bare-foot, even at home.

b) Do not cut your toenails too short and cut nails straight across.

RIGHT **WRONG**

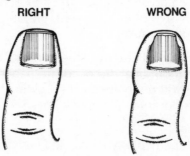

c) Never cut your own toenails if you have a significant eye-sight problem, or a nerve or blood vessel disorder affecting the feet: see a state-registered chiropodist regularly every 6–8 weeks if possible.

d) Avoid tight shoes: preferably have new shoes fitted by an expert who knows you are diabetic.

e) Wash, dry and examine your feet carefully at least every other day: even the most minor infection should be immediately discussed with your doctor.

f) Never attempt to treat any foot problem yourself. Permanent damage may result from the use of "over the counter" remedies: always seek professional advice first.

32. A FEW ADDITIONAL PROBLEMS

Can I smoke? Diabetes alone may damage the blood vessels of your body, as mentioned earlier. If you smoke as well your chances of such damage are that much greater.

Can I drive a car? Yes, but the licensing authorities may want to have your doctor's reassurance that your diabetes is sufficiently stable, and that you are otherwise well: an appropriate form will need to be completed, on which you must mention that you have diabetes.

Can I play sport as usual? Yes (see Questions 13 and 14).

Can I drink alcohol? Yes, but as mentioned earlier, calories do count. In addition, if you are prone to having many "hypos", alcohol (especially spirits) may block the body's corrective responses, and make your "hypos" more severe.

Does diabetes interfere with employment? No. Jobs involving physical responsibility for other people (eg bus drivers, airline pilots, certain branches of the armed forces), or involving personal danger (working on high buildings, diving etc) are not suitable for insulin-receiving diabetics. Apart from these situations, there should be no problems. The earlier discrimination against diabetics is now almost non-existent since it has been shown that the work record of diabetics is on average better than non-diabetics.

Can I get life insurance? Yes, you may have to accept a "loading", but life assurance is possible for most diabetics. Shop around and seek the advice of your Diabetic Association office.

Can I have children? Yes. Diabetes is at least partly inherited. If either parent is a diabetic the risk of any one child becoming diabetic at some time of their life is probably not more than two or three times the risk of any other person in the population.

Pregnancy in a diabetic should always be managed by a physician/obstetrician team accustomed to dealing with diabetic pregnancies: a lot of emphasis will be placed on making sure that your diabetes is well controlled. Your obstetrician may even wish you to spend the last few weeks of your pregnancy in hospital to ensure rest and the best possible control, and the baby may also be delivered a little earlier than usual.

Contraception Most of the presently available low-dose pills are satisfactory for diabetics and there is no reason why you cannot use intra-uterine devices (IUD) or other contraceptive methods. If you are planning a family, and especially if you are taking a contraceptive pill, let your doctor know. With your help, he will try to ensure that your control is as close as possible to perfection at the time you conceive. This is now considered to be important in reducing some problems which may occur in pregnancy. Once again, if you are "on the pill" it is useful to stop it and to have one normal period before you conceive, so that the exact stage of pregnancy is known. Your physicians will be happy to discuss other aspects of diabetes and pregnancy with you.

33. WHEN SHOULD I SEE MY DOCTOR?

Routinely

Ideally you should have a discussion with him or her at least every 3–4 months. Do not forget to take your test record book with you when you go.

At about yearly intervals and perhaps more frequently your doctor will systematically examine your eyes, blood pressure, heart, blood vessels on the feet and check for nerve damage. He will not mind if you remind him that your 12 months check is due. He might also take blood to see whether the blood fat (cholesterol and triglyceride) levels are normal, and may suggest an alteration to the diet if they are not.

As indicated earlier, a number of drugs in everyday use for other conditions may affect the control of your diabetes, or interfere with the dipstrip tests. Therefore, at these visits ask your doctor for reassurance that any of the other drugs that you are taking are not interfering in some way.

Each time you see either your family doctor or specialist, it is useful to take along your syringe (it may need checking), your diet sheet (it may need changing), and your urine or blood test record book (so that the doctor has information on which he may recommend any change in treatment).

45

In an Emergency

If you show heavy sugar consistently, or begin to feel thirsty or unwell do not wait: get advice. Make sure that you have one or more telephone numbers that you or your family or friends may contact for advice on such unexpected problems, and write them down in the space provided on page 47 (Question 37 "Hotline") for easy reference.

34. IDENTIFICATION

Always carry a card, or better still a bracelet or pendant, indicating that you are a diabetic. In this day and age accidents will happen, and it is obviously important that anyone can immediately identify you as being diabetic.

The Medicalert Foundation (local address available from your physician), which provides identification bracelets and pendants at a modest cost, now has branches in many countries. This system is highly recommended. Alternatively, have your local jeweller make up one for you.

35. FINALLY

Remember that knowing about your diabetes is your responsibility. Your physician, dietitian, clinic sister or chiropodist/podiatrist will be only too happy to answer queries and suggest further reading material.

Membership of your Diabetic Association has much to offer. It can help you follow recent trends in diabetes care. Much research is also being carried out in diabetes, including new methods of producing and giving insulin, and in transplanting the insulin-producing parts of the pancreas. You will find it useful and interesting to keep in touch with these and other important developments. If you are a youngster or teenager, diabetic associations provide group activities in which you may enjoy participating.

36. SOME ADDITIONAL READING

"Diabetes Explained" by Arnold Bloom, published by Medical and Technical Publications.

"Notes for the Guidance of Diabetic Children" by J.W. Farquhar, published by E.S. Livingstone.

"The Diabetic's Handbook" compiled by and obtainable from the British Diabetic Association.

"Living with Diabetes" by Helen Pond, MD, published by the British Diabetic Association.

"So your Child has Diabetes" by John Court, 2nd Edition 1978, Ure-Smith (Australia) – branch of Paul Hamlyn, London.

"The Diabetics Diet Book" by Jim Mann, Martin Dunitz, 1982.

37. "HOTLINE"

In this space a telephone number should be written from which you can get advice 24 hours a day, seven days a week should any sudden problem occur which affects your diabetes. Your doctor will advise you which number to insert.

....

38. OTHER IMPORTANT CONTACT NUMBERS

Your Family Doctor....................................

Your Diabetic Appointment Clerk..................

Your Dietitian...

Your Chiropodist..

Your Diabetic Advisory Service.....................

39. WHAT FOODS CAN I EAT?

Forbidden Foods

Some foods are very high in carbohydrate and in calories and must be excluded from your diet (unless you are actually treating a "hypo").

Sugar, jam, marmalade, honey, glucose
Sweet cakes and biscuits (especially those with jam or icing)
Sweetened drinks, squashes, for example Ribena and Lucozade
Sweets and chocolates.

Free Foods

The following have little or no carbohydrate, are low in calories, and can be taken freely.

SOUPS
Consomme, home-made soups (made from vegetables freely allowed), stock cubes, Oxo, Marmite, Bovril.

VEGETABLES
Artichokes, asparagus, aubergine, French beans, runner beans, beansprouts, broccoli, Brussels sprouts, cabbage, carrots, cauliflower, celeriac, celery, chicory, cucumber, endive, leeks, lettuce, marrow, courgettes, mushrooms, mustard and cress, okra, onions, parsley, peppers, pumpkin, radishes, salsify, seakale, spinach, spring greens, turnip, tomato, watercress.

FRUITS
Blackberries, blackcurrants, cranberries, redcurrants, gooseberries, grapefruit, lemon, loganberries, melon (all varieties), rhubarb.

DRINKS ETC

Tea, coffee (ground or instant), low calorie drinks labelled "Suitable for Diabetics", tomato juice, mineral waters, salt, pepper, herbs, spices, vinegar, Worcester sauce, saccharin in liquid or tablet form (not powder).

High Energy Foods

Other foods contain little or no carbohydrate, but are high in calories from fat or protein and therefore fattening. Watch these foods – particularly if you are overweight; eat in moderation. Avoid frying foods – try boiling, poaching, grilling or making casseroles.

Meat and poultry
Fish, eggs
Cheese – especially full-fat cheeses eg Cheddar
Butter, margarine, lard, dripping, all oils (including vegetable oils)
Cream
Diabetic sweets and chocolates.

Carbohydrate Exchange (portions)

All other foods containing carbohydrate are expressed as "exchanges" or "portions".

One exchange (or portion) = 10 grams of carbohydrate.

Do not confuse this with the actual weight of the food, which will be different – and always higher.

All the foods listed in the chart contain one exchange if eaten in the amount stated. You will be told how many exchanges to eat each day, and when during the day to eat them. It is important to eat the number of exchanges stated at the same time each day. If in doubt, ask your dietitian.

Those items shown in bold type are high in fibre.
Try to include as many of these as you can.

Carbohydrate Exchange List

BREAD

Bread (wholemeal)	1 medium slice	30g/1oz
Bread, Hovis or brown	1 small slice	20g/¾oz
Bread, white	1 small slice	20g/¾oz
Bread rolls (wholemeal)	½ small	20g/¾oz
Bread rolls, white	½ small	20g/¾oz
Bread, currant	1 small slice	20g/¾oz
Bread, malt	1 small slice	20g/¾oz
Bread, soda	1 small slice	20g/¾oz
Chappatis	1 thin	30g/1oz
Chappatis (wholemeal)	1 thin	30g/1oz

BISCUITS AND BAKED PRODUCTS

Ryvita	2	15g/½oz
Cream crackers	2	15g/½oz
Water biscuits	2	15g/½oz
Digestives	1 large or 2 small	15g/½oz
Matzo	3	15g/½oz
Semi-sweet (Rich Tea, Marie etc)	2	15g/½oz
Plain sponge cake (no jam)	Small piece	20g/¾oz
Pastry, flaky, cooked	1 tablespoon	25g/1oz
Pastry, shortcrust, cooked	1 tablespoon	20g/¾oz
Cornish pastie	small	45g/1½oz
Pizza, 12 cm	⅓	40g/1¼oz
Pork pie	individual	50g/1¾oz
Quiche	⅓ small	40g/1¼oz
Sausage roll (flaky pastry)	½ small	40g/1¼oz
Steak and kidney pie (individual cooked)	⅓	50g/1¾oz
Yorkshire pudding	1	50g/1¾oz

BREAKFAST CEREALS

All Bran	3 tablespoons	20g/¾oz
Branflakes	3 tablespoons	15g/½oz
Weetabix	1 biscuit	15g/½oz
Wheatflakes	3 tablespoons	15g/½oz
Wheatgerm	2 heaped tblspns	25g/1oz
Wheat bran	3 heaped tblspns	40g/1½oz
Shredded Wheat	1 biscuit	15g/½oz

Muesli	1 tablespoon	15g/½oz
Oatmeal	1 tablespoon	15g/½oz
Porridge (made with water)	4 tablespoons	120g/4¾oz
Ready Brek	1 tablespoon	15g/½oz
Puffed Wheat	3 tablespoons	15g/½oz
Cornflakes	3 tablespoons	15g/½oz
Rice Krispies	3 tablespoons	15g/½oz
Special K	3 tablespoons	15g/½oz

CEREALS

Pearl barley (raw)	1 tablespoon	10g/⅓oz
Pearl barley (cooked)	3 tablespoons	40g/1½oz
Flour (100% wholemeal)	1 level tblspn	15g/½oz
Flour, brown (85%)	1 tablespoon	15g/½oz
Flour, white	1 tablespoon	15g/½oz
Flour (100% rye)	1 tablespoon	15g/½oz
Cornflour/Custard powder	1 tablespoon	15g/½oz
Macaroni (raw, wholewheat)	1 tablespoon	15g/½oz
Macaroni (raw)	1 tablespoon	15g/½oz
Macaroni (boiled)	3 tablespoons	40g/1½oz
Noodles (raw)		15g/½oz
Rice (brown, raw)	1 tablespoon	15g/½oz
Rice (white, raw)	1 tablespoon	15g/½oz
Rice (white, boiled)	3 tablespoons	40g/1½oz
Sago (Tapioca, raw)	2 tablespoons	40g/1½oz
Semolina (wholewheat, raw)	2 tablespoons	15g/½oz
Semolina (raw)	2 tablespoons	15g/½oz
Spaghetti (wholewheat, raw)		15g/½oz
Spaghetti (raw)		15g/½oz
Spaghetti (boiled)	3 tablespoons	40g/1½oz
Spaghetti tinned in tomato sauce)		85g/3¼oz

DAIRY PRODUCTS

Milk, fresh whole	⅓ pint	200ml/8fl.oz
Milk, fresh skimmed	⅓ pint	200ml/8fl.oz
Milk, dried skimmed	2 tablespoons	20g/¾oz
Milk, evaporated	6 tablespoons	90ml/3fl.oz
Buttermilk	⅓ pint	200ml/8fl.oz
Yogurt, natural	1 carton	150g/5oz

Yogurt, fruit	½ small carton	60g/2oz
Ice-cream	1 brickette	50g/1¾oz

FRUIT

Apple (eating, skin and core)	1 medium size	120g/4oz
Apple (baked with skin)	1 medium	120g/4oz
Apple (stewed, no sugar)	6 level tblspns	120g/4oz
Apricots (fresh, with stones)	3	150g/6oz
Apricots (tinned in natural juice)	4 halves	180g/7oz
Banana (no skin)	½ medium	50g/1¾oz
Cherries (with stones)	20	100g/3½oz
Damsons (with stones)	3	120g/4oz
Grapes	10	60g/2oz
Grapefruit juice (unsweetened)	1 small glass	120ml/4fl.oz
Mandarin oranges (fresh only)	2	120g/4oz
Mandarin oranges (tinned in natural juice)	1 small tin	75g/2½oz
Mango, raw	2 tablespoons	60g/2oz
Nectarine (with stone)	1 medium	90g/3oz
Orange (fresh only)	1 medium	120g/4oz
Orange juice (unsweetened)	1 small glass	105ml/3½fl.oz
Papaya	1 medium slice	100g/4oz
Passion fruit	2 tablespoons	50g/2oz
Peach (with stone)	1 medium	120g/4oz
Pear (skin with core)	1 medium	120g/4oz
Pineapple (fresh)	1 large ring	90g/3oz
Pineapple (tinned in natural juice)	2 tablespoons	60g/2oz
Pineapple juice (unsweetened)	1 small glass	90ml/3fl.oz
Plums (with stones)	2	120g/4oz
Raspberries	7 tablespoons	180g/6oz
Strawberries	6 tablespoons	150g/5oz
Tangerine (fresh only)	2	120g/4oz
Prunes (dried, no stones)	3	25g/1oz

Dried fruit (currants, raisins, sultanas)	1 tablespoon	15g/½oz
Dates (dried with stones)	2	20g/¾oz
Figs (green, raw)	6	120g/4oz

MEAT AND FISH

Beefburger (frozen, raw)	2	240g/8oz
Beefburger (fried)	2	180g/6oz
Sausages (beef, raw)	2 large	90g/3oz
Sausages (beef, grilled)	2 large	60g/2oz
Sausages (pork, raw)	2 large	105g/3½oz
Sausages (pork, grilled)	2 large	90g/3oz
Fish cakes (fried)	1	60g/2oz
Fish fingers (fried)	3	60g/2oz

SOUPS

Cream of chicken (canned)	½ pint	200ml/10fl.oz
Chicken noodle (dried, as served)	½ pint	200ml/10fl.oz
Minestrone (dried, as served)	½ pint	200ml/10fl.oz
Cream of mushroom (canned)	½ pint	200ml/10fl.oz
Oxtail (canned)	1 large bowl	200ml/10fl.oz
Oxtail (dried, as served)	½ pint	200ml/10fl.oz
Tomato (dried, as served)	1 bowl	150ml/5fl.oz
Vegetable (canned)	1 bowl	150ml/5fl.oz

VEGETABLES AND BEANS

Baked beans in tomato sauce	4 tablespoons	120g/4oz
Butter beans (raw)	1 tablespoon	20g/¾oz
Butter beans (boiled)	3 tablespoons	60g/2oz
Chick peas (dried)	1 tablespoon	20g/¾oz
Chick peas (boiled)	2 tablespoons	45g/1½oz
Haricot beans (dried)	1 tablespoon	20g/¾oz
Haricot beans (boiled)	3 tablespoons	60g/2½oz
Lentils (raw)	1 tablespoon	20g/¾oz
Lentils (boiled)	3 tablespoons	60g/2oz

Mixed vegetables (frozen)	4 tablespoons	100g/4oz
Mungbeans (green gram, raw)	1 tablespoon	30g/1oz
Mungbeans (cooked)	3½ tablespoons	105g/3½oz
Parsnips (boiled)	3 tablespoons	90g/3oz
Peas (fresh, boiled)	5 tablespoons	150g/5oz
Peas (frozen, boiled)	9 tablespoons	240g/6oz
Peas (processed)	3 tablespoons	80g/2½oz
Peas (dried)	1 tablespoon	20g/¾oz
Peas (dried, boiled)	2 tablespoons	60g/2oz
Split peas (raw)	1 tablespoon	20g/¾oz
Split peas (boiled)	2 tablespoons	45g/1¾oz
Plantain (green, raw)	1 small piece	40g/1½oz
Plantain (boiled)	1 small piece	30g/1oz
Plantain (ripe, fried)	½ small piece	20g/¾oz
Potatoes (old, raw)	1 small (egg-size)	60g/2oz
Potatoes (old, boiled)	1 small (egg-size)	60g/2oz
Potatoes (baked)	1 small (egg-size)	60g/2oz
Potatoes (roast)	½ medium	40g/1½oz
Potatoes (chips)	4	30g/1oz
Potato chips (frozen, fried)	6	40g/1½oz
Potatoes (new, boiled)	1 small (egg-size)	60g/2oz
Potatoes (new, tinned)	1 medium	80g/2½oz
Potato, instant (made up)	2 tablespoons	60g/2oz
Potato crisps	1 small packet	20g/¾oz
Swede, raw		240g/8oz
Swede, boiled		240g/8oz
Sweetcorn (raw)	2 tablespoons	40g/1½oz
Sweetcorn (tinned)	2½ tablespoons	60g/2oz
Sweet potato (raw)	2 tablespoons	50g/1½oz
Sweet potato (boiled)	2 tablespoons	50g/1½oz
Yam (raw)	1 heaped tblspn	30g/1oz
Yam (boiled)	1 heaped tblspn	30g/1oz

ALCOHOL

Beer, draught mild	1 pint	550ml/20fl.oz
Beer, draught bitter	1 pint	550ml/20fl.oz
Lager, bottled	1¼ pint	650ml/25fl.oz
Pale ale, bottled	1 pint	550ml/20fl.oz
Stout, bottled	½ pint	280ml/10fl.oz
Cider, dry	¾ pint	450ml/15fl.oz

INDEX